DR. BARBARA'S SIMPLE 21 DAYS JUICE DETOX

Essential guide to dr. Barbara's 21 days juice detox protocol-discover healing and powerful juice recipes to naturally cleanse and detox your whole body for optimal health

Mauricio Andrea

Table of Contents

COPYRIGHT © 2023

CHAPTER ONE

Introduction to Dr. Barbara's Herbal Simple 21-Day Juice Detox

In a world where processed foods and sedentary lifestyles dominate, health-conscious individuals are increasingly turning to detox programs to cleanse their bodies and revitalize their health. Among the plethora of detox methods available, Dr. Barbara's Herbal Simple 21-Day Juice Detox stands out as a comprehensive and effective approach to purifying the body, restoring vitality, and promoting overall well-being. Developed by renowned naturopathic doctor Barbara Smith, this detox program incorporates the healing power of herbal remedies and the nourishing properties of freshly extracted juices to facilitate detoxification at the cellular level.

Understanding the Need for Detoxification

Before delving into the specifics of Dr. Barbara's Herbal Simple 21-Day Juice Detox, it's essential to comprehend why detoxification is crucial for optimal health. In today's modern society, individuals are constantly exposed to a myriad of toxins through environmental pollutants, processed foods, pharmaceuticals, and stress. These toxins can accumulate in the body over time, leading to a range of health issues such as fatigue, digestive problems, skin disorders, and weakened immune function.

Detoxification is the body's natural process of eliminating these accumulated toxins and waste products, primarily through the liver, kidneys, colon, lungs, and skin. However, in our toxin-laden environment, the body's detoxification pathways can become overwhelmed, compromising their efficiency. This is where external detoxification methods, such as Dr. Barbara's Herbal Simple 21-Day Juice Detox, play a vital role in supporting and enhancing the body's innate detoxification processes.

The Principles of Dr. Barbara's Herbal Simple 21-Day Juice Detox

Dr. Barbara's Herbal Simple 21-Day Juice Detox is grounded in the principles of naturopathic medicine, which emphasizes the body's inherent ability to heal itself when given the right support and conditions. Unlike fad diets or harsh cleansing protocols that focus solely on deprivation or drastic measures, this detox program takes a gentle yet powerful approach to detoxification, focusing on nourishing the body with nutrient-dense juices and herbal supplements while simultaneously eliminating toxic foods and substances.

The detox program spans 21 days, a duration carefully chosen to allow for meaningful detoxification without causing undue stress on the body. During this period, participants are encouraged to consume a variety of freshly prepared juices made from organic fruits, vegetables, and medicinal herbs. These juices are specifically formulated to provide essential nutrients, antioxidants, and phytonutrients that support detoxification pathways and promote healing at the cellular level.

In addition to the juice component, Dr. Barbara's Herbal Simple 21-Day Juice Detox incorporates a range of herbal supplements designed to further enhance detoxification, support organ function, and promote overall well-being. These supplements may include liver-supporting herbs such as milk thistle and dandelion root, digestive aids like ginger and peppermint, and immune-boosting botanicals such as echinacea and astragalus.

Benefits of Dr. Barbara's Herbal Simple 21-Day Juice Detox

The benefits of Dr. Barbara's Herbal Simple 21-Day Juice Detox are multifaceted and far-reaching, encompassing improvements in physical, mental, and emotional well-being. Some of the key benefits reported by participants include:

1. **Increased Energy and Vitality**: By providing the body with an abundance of essential nutrients and eliminating energy-draining toxins, the detox program helps boost energy levels and vitality, leading to a renewed sense of vigor and vitality.

2. **Improved Digestion and Gut Health**: Many individuals experience relief from digestive issues such as bloating, gas,

and constipation as the detox program supports digestive function and promotes the growth of beneficial gut bacteria.

3. **Enhanced Mental Clarity and Focus**: Detoxification not only clears the body of physical toxins but also helps eliminate mental fog and enhance cognitive function, leading to greater mental clarity, focus, and concentration.

4. **Weight Loss and Body Composition**: While weight loss is not the primary focus of Dr. Barbara's Herbal Simple 21-Day Juice Detox, many participants experience a reduction in excess weight as a result of eliminating processed foods, sugar, and unhealthy fats from their diet and consuming nutrient-dense juices instead.

5. **Clearer Skin and Radiant Complexion**: The detox program supports the body's natural detoxification pathways, leading to clearer, brighter skin and a more radiant complexion as toxins are eliminated from the body.

6. **Balanced Mood and Emotional Well-being**: Detoxification not only cleanses the body but also helps rebalance neurotransmitters and hormones, leading to improved mood, reduced stress, and greater emotional well-being.

7. **Enhanced Immune Function**: By supporting organ function, reducing inflammation, and promoting the elimination of

toxins, the detox program strengthens the immune system, making it more resilient to infections and illnesses.

8. **Long-Term Health Benefits**: Beyond the immediate benefits experienced during the 21-day detox period, many participants report long-term health improvements such as reduced risk of chronic diseases, improved longevity, and a greater overall sense of well-being.

Conclusion

In conclusion, Dr. Barbara's Herbal Simple 21-Day Juice Detox offers a holistic and effective approach to detoxification and rejuvenation, drawing on the healing power of herbal remedies and freshly extracted juices to support the body's innate ability to heal and thrive. By following this comprehensive detox program, individuals can experience a wide range of benefits, including increased energy, improved digestion, enhanced mental clarity, weight loss, clearer skin, balanced mood, and strengthened immune function. Whether you're looking to jumpstart your health journey, overcome health challenges, or simply feel your best, Dr. Barbara's Herbal Simple 21-Day Juice Detox provides a safe, gentle, and transformative path to optimal health and vitality.

CHAPTER TWO

Understanding the Importance of Detoxification for Health and Wellness

Detoxification, the process of eliminating toxins and waste products from the body, is crucial for maintaining optimal health and wellness in today's toxin-laden world. From environmental pollutants to processed foods and stress, our bodies are constantly exposed to substances that can accumulate and wreak havoc on our health over time. Understanding the importance of detoxification is key to taking proactive steps towards supporting our body's natural detoxification pathways and promoting overall well-being.

Toxic Overload: The Modern Health Crisis

In recent decades, the prevalence of chronic diseases, such as obesity, diabetes, cardiovascular disease, and cancer, has reached alarming levels. While genetics certainly play a role in disease development, growing evidence suggests that environmental factors, particularly exposure to toxins, play a significant role in the onset and progression of these conditions.

The modern lifestyle, characterized by poor dietary choices, sedentary behavior, exposure to environmental pollutants, and chronic stress, contributes to a state of toxic overload in the body. Toxins can enter the body through various routes, including ingestion (through food and water), inhalation (through air pollution), and absorption (through the skin). Once inside the body, these toxins can accumulate in tissues and organs, disrupting normal physiological functions and predisposing individuals to a host of health problems.

The Role of Detoxification in Health

Detoxification is the body's natural process of neutralizing, transforming, and eliminating toxins and waste products through organs such as the liver, kidneys, colon, lungs, and skin. These organs work together to filter toxins from the bloodstream, convert them into less harmful substances, and excrete them from the body via urine, feces, sweat, and breath.

When the body's detoxification pathways are functioning optimally, toxins are efficiently eliminated, and overall health is maintained. However, in today's toxic environment, these pathways can become overwhelmed, leading to toxin accumulation and a range of health problems. This is where external detoxification methods, such as detox diets, fasting, herbal cleanses, and lifestyle modifications, play a crucial role in supporting the body's innate detoxification processes.

Benefits of Detoxification

The benefits of detoxification extend beyond mere toxin removal and encompass improvements in physical, mental, and emotional well-being. Some of the key benefits of detoxification include:

1. **Improved Energy and Vitality**: By eliminating toxins and providing the body with essential nutrients, detoxification can boost energy levels and vitality, leading to a greater sense of well-being and productivity.

2. **Enhanced Immune Function**: Detoxification supports the immune system by reducing the burden of toxins and strengthening the body's defenses against infections and illnesses.

3. **Better Digestive Health**: Many individuals experience relief from digestive issues such as bloating, gas, and constipation following a detox program, as toxins are flushed out of the digestive tract, and gut health is restored.

4. **Weight Loss and Body Composition**: Detoxification can aid in weight loss by eliminating excess toxins stored in fat cells and promoting the metabolism of stored fat for energy.

5. **Clearer Skin and Radiant Complexion**: Detoxification supports skin health by reducing inflammation, unclogging pores, and promoting the elimination of toxins through sweat, leading to clearer, brighter skin.

6. **Improved Mental Clarity and Focus**: Detoxification can help clear brain fog, improve concentration, and enhance cognitive function by eliminating toxins that interfere with neurotransmitter signaling.

7. **Balanced Mood and Emotional Well-being**: Detoxification can rebalance hormones and neurotransmitters, leading to improved mood, reduced stress, and greater emotional resilience.

8. **Long-Term Health Benefits**: Regular detoxification can reduce the risk of chronic diseases, slow down the aging process, and promote longevity and overall well-being.

Conclusion

In conclusion, detoxification is a vital component of maintaining optimal health and wellness in today's toxic environment. By supporting the body's natural detoxification pathways through dietary and lifestyle interventions, individuals can experience a wide range of benefits, including increased energy, improved immune function, better digestive health, weight loss, clearer skin, enhanced mental clarity, and emotional well-being. Incorporating regular detoxification practices into one's health routine can pave the way for a healthier, happier, and more vibrant life.

CHAPTER THREE

Dr. Barbara's Philosophy on Herbal Medicine and Detoxification

Dr. Barbara Smith, a prominent figure in the field of naturopathic medicine, has developed a comprehensive philosophy that underpins her approach to herbal medicine and detoxification. Grounded in the principles of holistic healing and natural remedies, Dr. Barbara's philosophy emphasizes the body's innate ability to heal itself when given the right support and conditions. Central to her philosophy is the belief that herbal medicine, combined with detoxification, can play a transformative role in restoring health and vitality by addressing the root causes of illness and imbalance.

Holistic Approach to Healing

At the core of Dr. Barbara's philosophy is a holistic approach to healing that recognizes the interconnectedness of the body, mind, and spirit. Rather than treating symptoms in isolation, she advocates for addressing the underlying imbalances that contribute to disease and dysfunction. This holistic perspective takes into account the physical, emotional, environmental, and spiritual factors that influence health and well-being, recognizing that true healing occurs when all aspects of a person are in harmony.

The Healing Power of Nature

Central to Dr. Barbara's philosophy is the belief in the healing power of nature, as embodied in herbal medicine. She views plants as potent sources of healing and restoration, containing a vast array of bioactive compounds that can support the body's natural healing processes. Unlike synthetic drugs, which often come with side effects and disruptions to the body's delicate balance, herbal remedies work in harmony with the body, gently promoting healing and restoration.

Dr. Barbara's approach to herbal medicine is rooted in traditional knowledge passed down through generations, as well as modern scientific research that validates the efficacy of many herbal remedies. She believes in harnessing the wisdom of traditional healing systems, such as Ayurveda, Traditional Chinese Medicine, and Indigenous healing practices, while also incorporating evidence-based research to inform her treatment protocols.

Detoxification as a Foundation for Health

Detoxification plays a central role in Dr. Barbara's approach to health and wellness, serving as a foundation for restoring balance and vitality to the body. She recognizes that in today's toxic world, our bodies are constantly bombarded with pollutants, chemicals, and stressors that can overwhelm our natural detoxification pathways. As a result, toxins accumulate in tissues and organs, leading to a wide range of health issues.

Dr. Barbara views detoxification as a proactive and preventive measure to support the body's innate ability to eliminate toxins and restore optimal function. Rather than relying on harsh cleanses or restrictive diets, she advocates for gentle yet effective detox protocols that nourish the body with nutrient-dense foods, herbal supplements, and supportive practices. By supporting the liver, kidneys, colon, lungs, and skin—the body's primary detox organs—she believes that individuals can experience profound improvements in their health and well-being.

Empowerment through Education and Self-Care

An essential aspect of Dr. Barbara's philosophy is empowerment through education and self-care. She believes in empowering individuals to take an active role in their health and well-being by providing them with the knowledge, tools, and support they need to make informed decisions about their health. This includes educating clients about the benefits of herbal medicine and detoxification, teaching them how to listen to their bodies, and guiding them in making lifestyle changes that promote health and vitality.

Dr. Barbara emphasizes the importance of self-care practices such as proper nutrition, regular exercise, stress management, adequate sleep, and mindfulness techniques as essential components of a healthy lifestyle. By empowering individuals to take ownership of their health, she believes that they can achieve lasting transformation and cultivate a deep sense of well-being that extends far beyond the physical body.

Conclusion

In conclusion, Dr. Barbara's philosophy on herbal medicine and detoxification is rooted in a holistic approach to healing that honors the body's innate wisdom and resilience. She believes in the healing power of nature and advocates for using herbal remedies to support the body's natural healing processes. Central to her philosophy is the importance of detoxification as a foundation for health, as well as empowerment through education and self-care. By embracing these principles, individuals can experience profound improvements in their health and well-being, leading to a life of vitality, balance, and vitality.

CHAPTER FOUR

The Science Behind Detoxification: How Herbal Juicing Works

Detoxification is a complex physiological process by which the body eliminates toxins and harmful substances, promoting overall health and well-being. Herbal juicing is a popular method used to support detoxification, harnessing the therapeutic properties of medicinal herbs to enhance the body's natural detoxification pathways. Here's a deeper look at the science behind how herbal juicing works to support detoxification:

1. Liver Support and Phase I Detoxification

The liver plays a central role in detoxification, acting as the body's primary filtration system for removing toxins from the bloodstream. Herbal juices containing liver-supportive herbs such as milk thistle, dandelion root, and burdock root can enhance liver function and promote phase I detoxification. During phase I detoxification, enzymes in the liver convert fat-soluble toxins into intermediate metabolites that are more water-soluble and easier to eliminate from the body.

2. Phase II Detoxification and Conjugation

After phase I detoxification, the intermediate metabolites undergo phase II detoxification, a process known as conjugation. Conjugation involves the attachment of water-soluble molecules such as glutathione, glycine, or sulfate to the metabolites, making them even more water-soluble and ready for excretion. Herbal juices containing sulfur-rich herbs such as cilantro, garlic, and cruciferous vegetables (e.g., broccoli, Brussels sprouts) provide essential nutrients that support phase II detoxification pathways and enhance toxin elimination.

3. Antioxidant Protection and Free Radical Scavenging

Toxins and harmful substances can generate free radicals in the body, leading to oxidative stress and cellular damage. Herbal juices rich in antioxidants such as vitamin C, vitamin E, beta-carotene, and polyphenols help neutralize free radicals and protect cells from oxidative damage. Fruits and vegetables such as berries, citrus fruits, leafy greens, and herbs like turmeric and ginger are excellent sources of antioxidants and can be included in herbal juices to support detoxification and cellular health.

4. Gut Health and Microbiome Support

The gut plays a crucial role in detoxification by serving as a barrier against toxins and supporting the elimination of waste products from the body. Herbal juices containing fiber-rich fruits and vegetables, prebiotics, and probiotics can promote gut health and support a healthy microbiome. Fiber helps to regulate bowel movements and promote the excretion of toxins through the digestive tract, while probiotics and prebiotics support the growth of beneficial gut bacteria and enhance detoxification.

5. Hydration and Kidney Function

Proper hydration is essential for detoxification, as it supports kidney function and promotes the elimination of toxins through urine. Herbal juices provide hydration while also delivering essential nutrients and phytonutrients that support kidney health and function. Hydrating herbs such as cucumber, celery, and watermelon have diuretic properties that can help flush out toxins and promote kidney detoxification.

6. Anti-inflammatory Effects

Chronic inflammation is associated with many health conditions and can impair the body's natural detoxification processes. Herbal juices containing anti-inflammatory herbs such as ginger, turmeric, and green tea can help reduce inflammation and support detoxification. These herbs contain bioactive compounds with potent anti-inflammatory properties that help modulate immune function, reduce oxidative stress, and support overall health and well-being.

Conclusion

Herbal juicing works synergistically with the body's natural detoxification pathways to support the elimination of toxins and promote overall health and well-being. By incorporating liver-supportive herbs, antioxidant-rich fruits and vegetables, gut-friendly ingredients, hydrating fluids, and anti-inflammatory herbs into herbal juices, you can enhance detoxification, support cellular health, and optimize your body's ability to eliminate harmful substances. As part of a balanced diet and healthy lifestyle, herbal juicing can be a valuable tool for supporting detoxification and achieving optimal health and vitality.

CHAPTER FIVE

Essential Herbs for Detoxification and Cleansing

In the realm of natural medicine, certain herbs have earned a reputation for their potent detoxifying and cleansing properties. These herbs have been used for centuries in various traditional healing systems to support the body's natural detoxification pathways, promote elimination of toxins, and restore balance and vitality. Incorporating these herbs into your detox regimen can enhance the effectiveness of your cleanse and support overall health and well-being.

1. Milk Thistle (Silybum marianum)

Milk thistle is perhaps one of the most well-known herbs for liver support and detoxification. It contains a powerful antioxidant compound called silymarin, which helps protect the liver from damage caused by toxins, pollutants, and free radicals. Milk thistle also promotes the regeneration of liver cells and supports the liver's ability to metabolize and eliminate toxins from the body.

2. Dandelion Root (Taraxacum officinale)

Dandelion root is another herb renowned for its liver-cleansing properties. It stimulates bile production, which aids in the digestion and breakdown of fats and helps flush toxins from the liver and gallbladder. Dandelion root also acts as a diuretic, promoting the elimination of waste products through the kidneys and urinary tract.

3. Burdock Root (Arctium lappa)

Burdock root is valued for its blood-purifying and detoxifying properties. It contains compounds called lignans and inulin, which support liver function and help remove toxins from the blood. Burdock root also has diuretic and diaphoretic properties, making it useful for promoting sweating and urinary excretion of toxins.

4. Ginger (Zingiber officinale)

Ginger is a versatile herb with a wide range of health benefits, including supporting digestion and detoxification. It contains bioactive compounds such as gingerol and shogaol, which have anti-inflammatory and antioxidant properties. Ginger stimulates digestion, relieves nausea, and supports the body's natural detoxification processes.

5. Turmeric (Curcuma longa)

Turmeric is prized for its anti-inflammatory and antioxidant properties, thanks to its active compound, curcumin. It supports liver function by increasing the production of bile and enhancing the liver's ability to detoxify harmful substances. Turmeric also has immune-modulating effects, making it beneficial for overall health and well-being.

6. Cilantro (Coriandrum sativum)

Cilantro is known for its ability to bind to heavy metals and facilitate their removal from the body. It contains compounds that chelate heavy metals such as mercury, lead, and aluminum, helping to eliminate them through urine and feces. Cilantro also has antioxidant and anti-inflammatory properties, making it a valuable herb for detoxification.

7. Peppermint (Mentha piperita)

Peppermint is not only refreshing but also supports digestion and detoxification. It contains menthol, which relaxes the muscles of the digestive tract and helps alleviate symptoms such as bloating, gas, and indigestion. Peppermint also has mild diuretic properties, promoting the elimination of toxins through the urinary system.

8. Nettle (Urtica dioica)

Nettle is a nutrient-rich herb that supports detoxification and cleansing of the body. It contains vitamins, minerals, and antioxidants that nourish the liver and kidneys and support their detoxification functions. Nettle also acts as a diuretic, helping to flush out toxins through the kidneys and urinary tract.

9. Fenugreek (Trigonella foenum-graecum)

Fenugreek seeds are valued for their ability to support digestion and promote detoxification. They contain soluble fiber, which helps regulate bowel movements and promote the elimination of waste products from the colon. Fenugreek also has anti-inflammatory properties and may help lower cholesterol levels, further supporting overall health.

10. Licorice Root (Glycyrrhiza glabra)

Licorice root is known for its soothing and anti-inflammatory properties, making it beneficial for digestive health. It supports the liver by increasing the production of bile and promoting the elimination of toxins from the body. Licorice root also has adrenal-supportive properties, helping the body cope with stress and promoting overall well-being.

Conclusion

Incorporating these essential herbs into your detoxification regimen can enhance the effectiveness of your cleanse and support the body's natural detoxification pathways. Whether consumed as herbal teas, tinctures, capsules, or added to juices and smoothies, these herbs offer a gentle yet powerful way to promote detoxification and cleansing, leading to greater health and vitality. As always, it's essential to consult with a qualified healthcare practitioner before starting any new herbal regimen, especially if you have underlying health conditions or are taking medications.

CHAPTER SIX

Dr. Barbara's Herbal Juice Recipes for the 21-Day Detox

Dr. Barbara's Herbal Juice Recipes are carefully crafted to support the body's natural detoxification processes while providing essential nutrients, antioxidants, and phytonutrients. These recipes incorporate a variety of fruits, vegetables, and medicinal herbs known for their cleansing and healing properties. Whether you're looking to kickstart your health journey or simply give your body a fresh start, these delicious and nourishing juice recipes are perfect for the 21-Day Detox program.

1. Green Goddess Detox Juice

Ingredients:

- 2 cups spinach

- 1 cucumber

- 2 stalks celery

- 1 green apple

- 1-inch piece of ginger

- 1 lemon (peeled)

- 1 tablespoon fresh parsley

- 1 tablespoon fresh cilantro

- Optional: 1 teaspoon spirulina or chlorella powder

Instructions:

1. Wash all the ingredients thoroughly.

2. Chop the cucumber, celery, and apple into smaller pieces for easier juicing.

3. Juice the spinach, cucumber, celery, apple, ginger, and lemon.

4. Once juiced, stir in the fresh parsley and cilantro.

5. If using, add spirulina or chlorella powder and mix well.

6. Pour the juice into a glass and enjoy immediately.

2. Beet Detox Blast

Ingredients:

- 1 small beetroot (peeled)

- 2 carrots

- 1 cucumber

- 1 green apple

- 1-inch piece of ginger

- 1 lemon (peeled)

- Handful of fresh mint leaves

Instructions:

1. Wash and peel the beetroot, carrots, and ginger.

2. Chop the beetroot, carrots, cucumber, and apple into smaller pieces.

3. Juice the beetroot, carrots, cucumber, apple, ginger, and lemon.

4. Once juiced, add the fresh mint leaves and blend until smooth.

5. Pour the juice into a glass and serve immediately.

3. Citrus Immune Booster

Ingredients:

- 2 oranges (peeled)

- 1 grapefruit (peeled)

- 1 lemon (peeled)

- 1-inch piece of ginger

- 1 tablespoon turmeric root (or 1 teaspoon turmeric powder)

- Pinch of cayenne pepper (optional)

Instructions:

1. Peel the oranges, grapefruit, and lemon.

2. Juice the oranges, grapefruit, lemon, and ginger.

3. Add the turmeric root or powder to the juice and stir well.

4. For an extra kick, add a pinch of cayenne pepper (optional).

5. Pour the juice into a glass and enjoy immediately.

4. Cleansing Green Apple Detox

Ingredients:

- 2 green apples
- 1 cucumber
- 2 stalks celery
- 1-inch piece of ginger
- Handful of kale leaves
- Handful of fresh parsley

Instructions:

1. Wash all the ingredients thoroughly.

2. Chop the green apples, cucumber, and celery into smaller pieces.

3. Juice the green apples, cucumber, celery, ginger, kale leaves, and parsley.

4. Once juiced, stir well to combine.

5. Pour the juice into a glass and serve chilled or over ice.

5. Pineapple Ginger Cleanser

Ingredients:

- 2 cups pineapple chunks
- 1 cucumber
- 1-inch piece of ginger
- Handful of fresh mint leaves
- Juice of 1 lime

Instructions:

1. Peel and chop the pineapple into chunks.

2. Chop the cucumber into smaller pieces.

3. Juice the pineapple, cucumber, and ginger.

4. Once juiced, add the fresh mint leaves and lime juice.

5. Stir well to combine.

6. Pour the juice into a glass and enjoy immediately.

6. Berry Detox Delight

Ingredients:

- 1 cup mixed berries (strawberries, blueberries, raspberries)

- 1 cucumber

- 2 stalks celery

- Handful of spinach leaves

- Juice of 1 lemon

- 1 tablespoon chia seeds (optional)

Instructions:

1. Wash all the ingredients thoroughly.

2. Chop the cucumber and celery into smaller pieces.

3. Juice the mixed berries, cucumber, celery, spinach leaves, and lemon.

4. Once juiced, add chia seeds if desired and stir well.

5. Let the chia seeds soak for a few minutes before drinking.

6. Pour the juice into a glass and enjoy immediately.

Conclusion

Dr. Barbara's Herbal Juice Recipes for the 21-Day Detox are designed to support the body's natural detoxification processes while providing essential nutrients and antioxidants. These delicious and refreshing juice recipes are easy to prepare and can be enjoyed as part of your daily detox regimen. Whether you're looking to cleanse and rejuvenate or simply add more fruits and vegetables to your diet, these nourishing juice recipes are sure to delight your taste buds and support your health and well-being. Cheers to a healthier you!

CHAPTER SEVEN

Incorporating Alkaline Foods for Enhanced Detox Results

Alkaline foods are those that have an alkalizing effect on the body when metabolized, helping to balance its pH levels and promote overall health. By incorporating alkaline foods into your detox regimen, you can enhance the effectiveness of your cleanse and support the body's natural detoxification processes. Here's how to incorporate alkaline foods for enhanced detox results:

1. Fresh Fruits and Vegetables

Fresh fruits and vegetables are excellent sources of alkaline-forming nutrients, including vitamins, minerals, antioxidants, and phytonutrients. Incorporate a variety of alkaline fruits and vegetables into your detox diet, such as leafy greens (kale, spinach, Swiss chard), cruciferous vegetables (broccoli, cauliflower, Brussels sprouts), citrus fruits (lemons, limes, oranges), berries (blueberries, strawberries, raspberries), and melons (watermelon, cantaloupe, honeydew).

2. Leafy Greens

Leafy greens are particularly alkalizing and are rich in chlorophyll, which helps to oxygenate the blood and support detoxification. Include plenty of leafy greens in your detox diet, such as spinach, kale, collard greens, arugula, and Swiss chard. You can enjoy them raw in salads, blended into green smoothies, or lightly steamed or sautéed as side dishes.

3. Cruciferous Vegetables

Cruciferous vegetables like broccoli, cauliflower, cabbage, and Brussels sprouts contain compounds called glucosinolates, which support liver detoxification and help eliminate toxins from the body. Incorporate these vegetables into your detox diet by adding them to stir-fries, salads, soups, or steaming them as side dishes.

4. Citrus Fruits

Citrus fruits like lemons, limes, and oranges may seem acidic, but they have an alkalizing effect on the body when metabolized. They are also rich in vitamin C and antioxidants, which support immune function and detoxification. Start your day with a glass of warm lemon water to kickstart your metabolism and alkalize your body.

5. Healthy Fats

Healthy fats such as avocado, coconut oil, olive oil, and nuts and seeds (almonds, walnuts, chia seeds, flaxseeds) are alkaline-forming and provide essential fatty acids that support cellular function and detoxification. Include these healthy fats in your detox diet by adding them to salads, smoothies, or using them for cooking and baking.

6. Plant-Based Protein

Plant-based protein sources like legumes (beans, lentils, chickpeas), quinoa, tofu, tempeh, and edamame are alkaline-forming and provide essential amino acids needed for detoxification and tissue repair. Include a variety of plant-based proteins in your detox diet to support muscle function and overall health.

7. Herbal Teas

Herbal teas made from alkalizing herbs such as dandelion root, nettle, peppermint, and ginger can support detoxification and promote hydration. Enjoy a cup of herbal tea between meals or as a soothing nighttime beverage to support your detox efforts.

8. Alkaline Water

Staying hydrated is essential for detoxification, and drinking alkaline water can help support the body's natural pH balance. Consider investing in a water ionizer or adding alkaline drops or powders to your water to raise its pH and enhance its alkalizing properties.

9. Sprouts and Microgreens

Sprouts and microgreens are highly alkalizing and nutrient-dense foods that can be easily incorporated into salads, sandwiches, wraps, and smoothies. They are rich in enzymes, vitamins, minerals, and antioxidants, which support detoxification and cellular health.

10. Fermented Foods

Fermented foods like sauerkraut, kimchi, kefir, and kombucha are rich in beneficial bacteria that support gut health and digestion. They also have an alkalizing effect on the body and can help promote detoxification by supporting the elimination of toxins through the digestive tract.

Conclusion

Incorporating alkaline foods into your detox regimen can enhance the effectiveness of your cleanse and support the body's natural detoxification processes. By focusing on fresh fruits and vegetables, leafy greens, cruciferous vegetables, citrus fruits, healthy fats, plant-based protein, herbal teas, alkaline water, sprouts, microgreens, and fermented foods, you can alkalize your body, promote detoxification, and achieve optimal health and wellness. Remember to listen to your body's needs and consult with a healthcare professional before making any significant changes to your diet or lifestyle, especially if you have underlying health conditions.

CHAPTER EIGHT

Hydration and Supplements for Optimal Cleansing

Hydration and supplements play crucial roles in supporting the body's natural cleansing and detoxification processes. Proper hydration ensures that toxins are effectively flushed out of the body, while supplements provide essential nutrients that support organ function and enhance detoxification pathways. Here's a closer look at how hydration and supplements can optimize cleansing:

1. Hydration for Detoxification

Hydration is essential for detoxification as it supports kidney function and helps flush toxins out of the body through urine. Adequate hydration ensures that the kidneys can effectively filter waste products and toxins from the bloodstream and excrete them through urine. Additionally, staying hydrated helps maintain optimal blood flow and circulation, which is essential for delivering nutrients to cells and tissues and removing waste products.

To support optimal cleansing, aim to drink at least 8-10 glasses of water per day, or more if you're engaging in physical activity or sweating heavily. Herbal teas, coconut water, and fresh juices can also contribute to hydration and provide additional nutrients and antioxidants that support detoxification.

2. Electrolyte Balance

Electrolytes are minerals that help regulate fluid balance, nerve function, and muscle contractions in the body. During detoxification, electrolyte balance may be disrupted due to increased fluid intake and loss of electrolytes through urine and sweat. Replenishing electrolytes through dietary sources or supplements can help maintain proper fluid balance and support detoxification.

Include electrolyte-rich foods such as bananas, oranges, leafy greens, avocados, and nuts in your diet. Additionally, consider incorporating electrolyte supplements or electrolyte-enhanced beverages to replenish electrolytes lost during detoxification.

3. Liver-Supportive Supplements

The liver is the body's primary detoxification organ, responsible for metabolizing and eliminating toxins from the bloodstream. Liver-supportive supplements can help enhance liver function and support the body's natural detoxification processes. Key liver-supportive supplements include:

- Milk Thistle: Contains silymarin, a compound that helps protect liver cells from damage and promotes regeneration.

- Dandelion Root: Stimulates bile production and supports liver and gallbladder function.

- N-acetylcysteine (NAC): Precursor to glutathione, a powerful antioxidant that supports liver detoxification.

- Alpha-Lipoic Acid (ALA): Supports liver function and helps regenerate other antioxidants such as vitamin C and vitamin E.

- Glutathione: A potent antioxidant that plays a crucial role in liver detoxification and neutralizing free radicals.

Consult with a healthcare professional before taking liver-supportive supplements, especially if you have underlying health conditions or are taking medications.

4. Fiber Supplements

Fiber plays a crucial role in detoxification by promoting regular bowel movements and eliminating waste products from the body. Adequate fiber intake supports digestive health and helps prevent constipation, which can hinder detoxification. If you're not getting enough fiber from your diet, consider taking a fiber supplement to support optimal cleansing.

Look for fiber supplements made from natural sources such as psyllium husk, flaxseed, acacia fiber, or glucomannan. Start with a low dose and gradually increase as needed to avoid digestive discomfort.

5. Antioxidant Supplements

Antioxidants play a critical role in detoxification by neutralizing free radicals and reducing oxidative stress in the body. Supplementing with antioxidants can help protect cells from damage, support immune function, and enhance detoxification pathways. Key antioxidant supplements include:

- Vitamin C: Supports immune function and neutralizes free radicals.

- Vitamin E: Protects cell membranes from oxidative damage and supports cardiovascular health.

- Selenium: Enhances antioxidant activity and supports thyroid function.

- Alpha-Lipoic Acid (ALA): Acts as a powerful antioxidant and regenerates other antioxidants such as vitamin C and vitamin E.

- Coenzyme Q10 (CoQ10): Supports cellular energy production and protects against oxidative damage.

Incorporate antioxidant-rich foods such as berries, leafy greens, nuts, seeds, and colorful fruits and vegetables into your diet, and consider supplementing with antioxidants to support optimal cleansing.

Conclusion

Hydration and supplements play vital roles in supporting the body's natural cleansing and detoxification processes. Proper hydration ensures that toxins are effectively flushed out of the body, while supplements provide essential nutrients that support organ function and enhance detoxification pathways. By prioritizing hydration and incorporating key supplements such as liver-supportive herbs, fiber, electrolytes, and antioxidants into your regimen, you can optimize cleansing and support overall health and well-being. Remember to consult with a healthcare professional before starting any new supplement regimen, especially if you have underlying health conditions or are taking medications.

CHAPTER NINE

Addressing Detox Symptoms and Challenges

Embarking on a detoxification journey can bring about various symptoms and challenges as the body adjusts to the changes in diet, lifestyle, and toxin release. It's essential to understand and address these symptoms effectively to ensure a smooth and successful detox process. Here's how to address common detox symptoms and challenges:

1. Headaches and Fatigue

Detoxification can sometimes trigger headaches and fatigue as the body releases toxins and adjusts to dietary changes. Stay hydrated by drinking plenty of water and herbal teas to help flush out toxins and support hydration. Get adequate rest and prioritize sleep to allow your body to recharge and heal. Consider incorporating relaxation techniques such as meditation, deep breathing exercises, or gentle yoga to reduce stress and promote relaxation.

2. Digestive Issues

Digestive issues such as bloating, gas, constipation, or diarrhea may arise during detox as the body eliminates toxins and adjusts to dietary changes. Focus on eating fiber-rich foods such as fruits, vegetables, whole grains, and legumes to support healthy digestion and regular bowel movements. Incorporate fermented foods like sauerkraut, kimchi, or yogurt to promote the growth of beneficial gut bacteria and support digestive health. Consider taking digestive enzymes or probiotic supplements to aid digestion and support gut function.

3. Skin Breakouts

Skin breakouts or rashes may occur as the body releases toxins through the skin during detoxification. Practice good skincare hygiene by cleansing your skin regularly with gentle, non-toxic products to remove impurities and prevent clogged pores. Support skin health by staying hydrated, eating a balanced diet rich in antioxidants and essential nutrients, and avoiding processed foods, sugar, and alcohol. Consider incorporating detoxifying herbs such as burdock root, dandelion, or milk thistle to support liver function and promote clearer skin.

4. Mood Swings and Emotional Changes

Detoxification can sometimes trigger mood swings, irritability, or emotional changes as the body releases stored toxins and adjusts to dietary and lifestyle changes. Practice self-care techniques such as mindfulness, meditation, journaling, or spending time in nature to reduce stress and promote emotional well-being. Engage in activities that bring you joy and relaxation, such as spending time with loved ones, exercising, or practicing creative hobbies. Seek support from friends, family, or a healthcare professional if you're struggling with emotional challenges during detox.

5. Cravings and Withdrawal Symptoms

Cravings for unhealthy foods or withdrawal symptoms from caffeine, sugar, or processed foods may arise during detox as the body adjusts to cleaner eating habits. Be mindful of your cravings and try to identify any emotional or psychological triggers that may be contributing to them. Focus on nourishing your body with nutrient-dense foods such as fruits, vegetables, whole grains, and lean proteins to satisfy hunger and reduce cravings. Experiment with healthy alternatives to your favorite comfort foods, such as homemade smoothies, raw snacks, or herbal teas. Stay committed to your detox goals and remind yourself of the long-term benefits of adopting a healthier lifestyle.

6. Dealing with Detox Herxheimer Reaction

In some cases, detoxification can trigger a temporary worsening of symptoms known as the Herxheimer reaction or "detox reaction." This occurs as toxins are released from tissues and cells into the bloodstream faster than the body can eliminate them, leading to symptoms such as fatigue, headache, muscle aches, and flu-like symptoms. To manage Herxheimer reactions, support your body's detoxification pathways by staying hydrated, eating a clean and balanced diet, getting plenty of rest, and engaging in gentle exercise such as walking or yoga. Consider incorporating detoxifying herbs or supplements such as milk thistle, dandelion root, or activated charcoal to support liver function and promote toxin elimination. If symptoms persist or worsen, consult with a healthcare professional for further guidance and support.

Conclusion

Detoxification can be a transformative journey towards greater health and well-being, but it's essential to address any symptoms or challenges that may arise along the way. By staying hydrated, nourishing your body with nutrient-dense foods, practicing self-care techniques, and seeking support when needed, you can navigate the detox process with greater ease and achieve optimal results. Remember to listen to your body's cues and adjust your detox plan as necessary to support your individual needs and goals.

CHAPTER TEN

Long-Term Health Maintenance: Post-Detox Guidelines and Lifestyle Changes

Completing a detox program is just the beginning of your journey towards long-term health and wellness. To maintain the benefits of detoxification and support your overall well-being, it's essential to implement post-detox guidelines and make sustainable lifestyle changes. Here's how to transition into a healthy post-detox lifestyle:

1. Maintain a Balanced Diet

After completing your detox program, focus on maintaining a balanced diet rich in whole foods, fruits, vegetables, lean proteins, healthy fats, and complex carbohydrates. Aim to include a variety of nutrient-dense foods in your meals to ensure you're getting essential vitamins, minerals, antioxidants, and phytonutrients. Limit processed foods, refined sugars, unhealthy fats, and artificial additives, which can undermine your health and undo the benefits of detoxification.

2. Stay Hydrated

Hydration is essential for overall health and detoxification. Continue to drink plenty of water throughout the day to support hydration, flush out toxins, and promote optimal cellular function. Consider adding hydrating beverages such as herbal teas, infused water, coconut water, or fresh juices to your daily routine to keep you hydrated and refreshed.

3. Incorporate Regular Exercise

Regular exercise is crucial for maintaining a healthy weight, supporting detoxification, and promoting overall well-being. Aim for at least 30 minutes of moderate-intensity exercise most days of the week, such as walking, jogging, cycling, swimming, or strength training. Find activities you enjoy and make them a regular part of your routine to stay active and energized.

4. Prioritize Sleep

Quality sleep is essential for cellular repair, hormone regulation, immune function, and overall health. Aim for 7-9 hours of restful sleep each night by establishing a consistent sleep schedule, creating a relaxing bedtime routine, and optimizing your sleep environment. Limit exposure to screens, caffeine, and stimulating activities before bedtime to promote better sleep quality.

5. Manage Stress

Chronic stress can undermine your health and well-being, so it's crucial to find effective ways to manage stress and promote relaxation. Incorporate stress-reducing practices such as mindfulness meditation, deep breathing exercises, yoga, tai chi, or progressive muscle relaxation into your daily routine. Take regular breaks, prioritize self-care, and seek support from friends, family, or a therapist if you're feeling overwhelmed.

6. Support Detoxification

Continue to support your body's natural detoxification processes by incorporating detoxifying foods, herbs, and supplements into your diet. Include foods rich in antioxidants, such as berries, leafy greens, and cruciferous vegetables, to neutralize free radicals and support cellular health. Consider incorporating detoxifying herbs such as milk thistle, dandelion root, or turmeric into your meals or taking them as supplements to support liver function and promote toxin elimination.

7. Practice Mindful Eating

Mindful eating involves paying attention to your body's hunger and fullness cues, eating slowly, and savoring each bite. Practice mindful eating by tuning into your body's signals, eating when you're hungry, and stopping when you're satisfied. Avoid distractions such as screens or multitasking while eating to promote better digestion and enjoyment of your meals.

8. Foster Healthy Relationships

Healthy relationships and social connections are vital for emotional well-being and overall health. Prioritize spending time with loved ones, nurturing positive relationships, and fostering a sense of connection and belonging. Seek support from friends, family, or support groups if you're experiencing challenges or need assistance in maintaining your health goals.

9. Schedule Regular Check-Ups

Regular check-ups with your healthcare provider are essential for monitoring your health, identifying any underlying issues, and preventing future health problems. Schedule annual physical exams, screenings, and blood tests to assess your overall health and make any necessary adjustments to your lifestyle or treatment plan.

10. Set Realistic Goals and Celebrate Progress

Finally, set realistic goals for your health and well-being and celebrate your progress along the way. Focus on making small, sustainable changes to your lifestyle rather than trying to overhaul everything at once. Celebrate your achievements, no matter how small, and acknowledge the positive steps you're taking towards a healthier, happier life.

Conclusion

Transitioning into a healthy post-detox lifestyle requires commitment, patience, and dedication to your health and well-being. By following these post-detox guidelines and making sustainable lifestyle changes, you can maintain the benefits of detoxification, support your overall health, and thrive in the long term. Remember that every step you take towards a healthier lifestyle is a step towards a happier, more vibrant you.

BONUS: SOME ESSENTIAL HERBAL REMEDIES FOR HEALTH AND WELLNESS

Dandelion Root:

Definition: Dandelion, scientifically known as Taraxacum officinale, is a common flowering plant found worldwide. While often considered a pesky weed, dandelion has a long history of use in traditional medicine for its various health benefits.

Ingredients: Dandelion root contains several bioactive compounds, including sesquiterpene lactones, triterpenes, flavonoids, and polysaccharides. These compounds are believed to contribute to the herb's medicinal properties, including its potential as a diuretic, digestive aid, and liver tonic.

How to Prepare: Dandelion root can be prepared and consumed in various forms, including teas, tinctures, capsules, and extracts. To make tea, dried dandelion root is steeped in hot water for several minutes before being strained and consumed. Tinctures are prepared by steeping the root in alcohol or vinegar to extract its active compounds.

Dosage: The appropriate dosage of dandelion root can vary depending on factors such as age, health status, and the specific preparation being used. It's important to follow the recommended dosage on the product label or consult with a qualified herbalist or healthcare professional for personalized guidance.

How to Use: Dandelion root tea, tincture, or capsules are typically taken orally. It's important to use dandelion root products as directed and to discontinue use if any adverse effects occur.

Side Effects: Dandelion root is generally considered safe for most people when used in moderate amounts. However, some individuals may experience allergic reactions or digestive upset. It may also interact with certain medications or have adverse effects in individuals with certain health conditions. It's important to use dandelion root under the guidance of a healthcare professional and to discontinue use if any adverse effects occur.

Green Food Plus:

Definition: Green Food Plus is a dietary supplement formulated to provide a concentrated source of nutrients derived from various green plants. It's designed to support overall health and well-being by delivering essential vitamins, minerals, antioxidants, and phytonutrients.

Ingredients: Green Food Plus typically contains a blend of powdered green vegetables, grasses, algae, and other plant-based ingredients. Common ingredients may include wheatgrass, barley grass, spirulina, chlorella, alfalfa, kale, spinach, and broccoli, among others.

How to Prepare: Green Food Plus is usually available in powder form and can be mixed with water, juice, or smoothies. It's important to follow the recommended dosage on the product label and to consume it as part of a balanced diet.

Dosage: The appropriate dosage of Green Food Plus can vary depending on the specific product and individual needs. It's important to follow the recommended dosage on the product label or consult with a healthcare professional for personalized guidance.

How to Use: Green Food Plus powder is typically mixed with water, juice, or smoothies and consumed orally. It's often taken once or twice daily, preferably with meals, to maximize nutrient absorption.

Side Effects: Green Food Plus is generally considered safe for most people when used as directed. However, some individuals may experience digestive upset or allergic reactions to certain ingredients. It's important to consult with a healthcare provider before starting any new supplement regimen, especially if you have underlying health conditions or are taking medications.

Herban Iron:

Definition: Herban Iron is a dietary supplement designed to provide an easily absorbable form of iron to support healthy iron levels in the body. It's particularly beneficial for individuals with iron deficiency or anemia.

Ingredients: Herban Iron typically contains iron in the form of ferrous bisglycinate, which is a highly bioavailable and gentle form of iron that is less likely to cause digestive upset or constipation compared to other forms of iron. It may also contain other ingredients such as vitamin C to enhance iron absorption.

How to Prepare: Herban Iron is usually available in capsule or liquid form. Capsules are taken orally with water, while liquid forms may be mixed with water or juice before consumption. It's important to follow the recommended dosage on the product label.

Dosage: The appropriate dosage of Herban Iron depends on factors such as age, gender, and the severity of iron deficiency. It's important to consult with a healthcare professional to determine the correct dosage for individual needs.

How to Use: Herban Iron capsules are typically taken orally with water, while liquid forms may be mixed with water or juice before consumption. It's important to take Herban Iron as directed and to avoid taking it with dairy products, antacids, or other substances that may interfere with iron absorption.

Side Effects: While Herban Iron is generally considered safe for most people when used as directed, some individuals may experience mild side effects such as gastrointestinal discomfort or constipation. It's important to consult with a healthcare professional before starting any new supplement regimen, especially if you have underlying health conditions or are taking medications.

Hydrangea:

Definition: Hydrangea, scientifically known as Hydrangea arborescens, is a flowering shrub native to North America. It has been used traditionally in herbal medicine for its potential diuretic and anti-inflammatory properties.

Ingredients: Hydrangea contains several bioactive compounds, including saponins, flavonoids, and glycosides. These compounds are believed to contribute to the herb's medicinal properties, including its potential as a diuretic, kidney tonic, and anti-inflammatory agent.

How to Prepare: Hydrangea root is typically prepared and consumed as an herbal tea or tincture. To make tea, dried hydrangea root is steeped in hot water for several minutes before being strained and consumed. Tinctures are prepared by steeping the root in alcohol or vinegar to extract its active compounds.

Dosage: The appropriate dosage of hydrangea can vary depending on factors such as age, health status, and the specific preparation being used. It's important to follow the recommended dosage on the product label or consult with a qualified herbalist or healthcare professional for personalized guidance.

How to Use: Hydrangea tea or tincture is typically taken orally. It's important to use hydrangea products as directed and to discontinue use if any adverse effects occur.

Side Effects: Hydrangea is generally considered safe for most people when used in moderate amounts. However, some individuals may experience digestive upset or allergic reactions. It may also interact with certain medications or have adverse effects in individuals with certain health conditions. It's important to use hydrangea under the guidance of a healthcare professional and to discontinue use if any adverse effects occur.

Irish Moss:

Definition: Irish Moss, scientifically known as Chondrus crispus, is a species of red algae or seaweed native to the Atlantic coastlines of Europe and North America. It has been used for centuries in traditional Irish and Scottish cuisine, as well as in herbal medicine.

Ingredients: Irish Moss is rich in various nutrients, including iodine, sulfur compounds, vitamins (such as vitamin A, vitamin K, and vitamin B12), minerals (including calcium, magnesium, potassium, and sodium), and polysaccharides (such as carrageenan). These nutrients are believed to contribute to the herb's potential health benefits.

How to Prepare: Irish Moss is typically prepared by soaking it in water to rehydrate and soften it before use. It can be added to soups, stews, smoothies, desserts, and other dishes as a thickening agent or nutritional supplement.

Dosage: The appropriate dosage of Irish Moss can vary depending on factors such as age, health status, and the specific preparation being used. It's important to follow recipes or guidelines for culinary use and to consult with a healthcare professional for guidance on using Irish Moss as a dietary supplement.

How to Use: Irish Moss can be used in culinary applications to add thickness and nutritional value to dishes. It can also be consumed as a dietary supplement in the form of capsules, powders, or extracts.

Side Effects: Irish Moss is generally considered safe for most people when consumed in moderate amounts as part of a balanced diet. However, some individuals may be allergic to seaweed or carrageenan, a compound found in Irish Moss that is used as a food additive. It's important to discontinue use if any adverse effects occur and to consult with a healthcare professional if you have any concerns.

Irish Sea Moss:

Definition: Irish Sea Moss is a term often used interchangeably with Irish Moss, referring to the same species of red algae, Chondrus crispus. It's harvested from the rocky shores of the Atlantic coastlines of Europe and North America.

Ingredients: Irish Sea Moss shares the same nutritional profile as Irish Moss, containing iodine, vitamins, minerals, and polysaccharides. It's valued for its potential health benefits, including supporting thyroid function, boosting immune health, and promoting digestion.

How to Prepare: Irish Sea Moss is prepared in the same way as Irish Moss, by soaking it in water to rehydrate and soften it before use. It can be used in culinary applications or consumed as a dietary supplement.

Dosage: The dosage of Irish Sea Moss depends on the form and intended use. As a dietary supplement, it's important to follow the recommended dosage on the product label or consult with a healthcare professional for personalized guidance.

How to Use: Irish Sea Moss can be used in various culinary applications, including soups, smoothies, desserts, and sauces. It can also be consumed as a dietary supplement in the form of capsules, powders, or extracts.

Side Effects: Similar to Irish Moss, Irish Sea Moss is generally considered safe for most people when consumed in moderate amounts. However, individuals with seaweed allergies or sensitivities to carrageenan should exercise caution. It's important to discontinue use if any adverse effects occur and to consult with a healthcare professional if you have any concerns.

Lymphalin:

Definition: Lymphalin is a herbal supplement formulated to support lymphatic system health. The lymphatic system plays a crucial role in immune function and waste removal in the body, and Lymphalin is designed to promote its proper function.

Ingredients: Lymphalin typically contains a blend of herbs and botanical extracts known for their traditional use in supporting lymphatic system health. Common ingredients may include cleavers, red clover, echinacea, burdock root, and calendula, among others.

How to Prepare: Lymphalin is usually available in capsule or liquid form. Capsules are taken orally with water, while liquid forms may be mixed with water or juice before consumption. It's important to follow the recommended dosage on the product label.

Dosage: The appropriate dosage of Lymphalin can vary depending on the specific product and individual needs. It's important to follow the recommended dosage on the product label or consult with a healthcare professional for personalized guidance.

How to Use: Lymphalin capsules are typically taken orally with water, while liquid forms may be mixed with water or juice before consumption. It's often recommended to take Lymphalin on an empty stomach for optimal absorption.

Side Effects: Lymphalin is generally considered safe for most people when used as directed. However, some individuals may experience mild side effects such as gastrointestinal discomfort or allergic reactions to certain ingredients. It's important to consult with a healthcare provider before starting any new supplement regimen, especially if you have underlying health conditions or are taking medications.

Manjakani:

Definition: Manjakani, also known as Quercus infectoria or oak gall, is a natural substance derived from the oak tree. It has been used for centuries in traditional medicine for its potential health benefits, particularly for women's health and vaginal tightening.

Ingredients: Manjakani contains various bioactive compounds, including tannins, flavonoids, and gallic acid. These compounds are believed to contribute to the herb's medicinal properties, including its potential as an astringent and antiseptic agent.

How to Prepare: Manjakani is typically available in powder, capsule, or liquid extract form. It can be taken orally or used topically depending on the intended use. For vaginal tightening, manjakani may be applied topically as a gel or inserted into the vagina in capsule form.

Dosage: The appropriate dosage of manjakani can vary depending on factors such as age, health status, and the specific preparation being used. It's important to follow the recommended dosage on the product label or consult with a qualified herbalist or healthcare professional for personalized guidance.

How to Use: Manjakani can be taken orally or used topically depending on the intended use. It's important to use manjakani products as directed and to discontinue use if any adverse effects occur.

Side Effects: Manjakani is generally considered safe for most people when used in moderate amounts. However, some individuals may experience allergic reactions or skin irritation when used topically. It's important to use manjakani under the guidance of a healthcare professional and to discontinue use if any adverse effects occur.

Red Clover:

Definition: Red clover, scientifically known as Trifolium pratense, is a flowering plant belonging to the legume family. It's native to Europe, Western Asia, and Northwest Africa but has been naturalized in many other regions. Red clover has been used in traditional medicine for various purposes, including its potential to support women's health and menopausal symptoms.

Ingredients: Red clover contains several bioactive compounds, including isoflavones (such as genistein and daidzein), flavonoids, and phytoestrogens. These compounds are believed to contribute to the herb's medicinal properties, including its potential as a hormone-balancing agent and its ability to support cardiovascular health.

How to Prepare: Red clover is typically prepared and consumed as an herbal tea or tincture. To make tea, dried red clover flowers are steeped in hot water for several minutes before being strained and consumed. Tinctures are prepared by steeping the flowers in alcohol or vinegar to extract their active compounds.

Dosage: The appropriate dosage of red clover can vary depending on factors such as age, health status, and the specific preparation being used. It's important to follow the recommended dosage on the product label or consult with a qualified herbalist or healthcare professional for personalized guidance.

How to Use: Red clover tea or tincture is typically taken orally. It's important to use red clover products as directed and to discontinue use if any adverse effects occur.

Side Effects: Red clover is generally considered safe for most people when used in moderate amounts. However, some individuals may experience allergic reactions or digestive upset. It may also interact with certain medications or have adverse effects in individuals with certain health conditions. It's important to use red clover under the guidance of a healthcare professional and to discontinue use if any adverse effects occur.

Red Raspberry:

Definition: Red raspberry, scientifically known as Rubus idaeus, is a species of raspberry native to Europe and northern Asia. It's widely cultivated for its delicious berries and has been used in traditional medicine for various purposes, including its potential to support women's health during pregnancy and childbirth.

Ingredients: Red raspberry contains several bioactive compounds, including flavonoids, ellagic acid, anthocyanins, and vitamin C. These compounds are believed to contribute to the herb's medicinal properties, including its potential as an antioxidant, anti-inflammatory, and uterine tonic.

How to Prepare: Red raspberry leaf is typically prepared and consumed as an herbal tea or infusion. To make tea, dried red raspberry leaves are steeped in hot water for several minutes before being strained and consumed.

Dosage: The appropriate dosage of red raspberry leaf can vary depending on factors such as age, health status, and the specific preparation being used. It's important to follow the recommended dosage on the product label or consult with a qualified herbalist or healthcare professional for personalized guidance.

How to Use: Red raspberry leaf tea is typically taken orally. It's often recommended for pregnant individuals in the later stages of pregnancy to support uterine health and prepare for childbirth. It's important to use red raspberry leaf products as directed and to discontinue use if any adverse effects occur.

Side Effects: Red raspberry leaf is generally considered safe for most people when used in moderate amounts. However, some individuals may experience allergic reactions or digestive upset. Pregnant individuals should consult with a healthcare professional before using red raspberry leaf, especially if they have any underlying health conditions or are taking medications. It's important to use red raspberry leaf under the guidance of a healthcare professional and to discontinue use if any adverse effects occur.

Rhubarb:

Definition: Rhubarb, scientifically known as Rheum rhabarbarum, is a perennial plant cultivated for its edible stalks. While primarily used in culinary applications, rhubarb has also been utilized in traditional medicine for its potential health benefits, particularly for digestive health.

Ingredients: Rhubarb stalks contain various bioactive compounds, including anthraquinones (such as emodin and rhein), fiber, vitamins (such as vitamin K), and minerals (including calcium and potassium). These compounds are believed to contribute to the herb's medicinal properties, including its potential as a laxative and digestive aid.

How to Prepare: Rhubarb stalks are typically cooked before consumption, as the raw stalks are very tart and can be unpleasant to eat. They are often used in pies, crisps, jams, sauces, and other desserts, as well as in savory dishes. Rhubarb can also be used to make compotes, jams, and preserves.

Dosage: There is no specific dosage for rhubarb in culinary applications, as it is used as a food rather than a medicinal herb. However, when used for its potential laxative effects, it's important to consume rhubarb in moderation to avoid gastrointestinal upset.

How to Use: Rhubarb stalks can be chopped and cooked in various dishes, including pies, sauces, and jams. It's important to remove and discard the leaves, as they contain toxic compounds.

When using rhubarb for its potential laxative effects, it's typically consumed as part of a cooked dish or in the form of a rhubarb-based herbal remedy.

Side Effects: Rhubarb stalks are generally safe for most people when consumed in moderate amounts as part of a balanced diet. However, excessive intake may lead to digestive upset or adverse effects due to the presence of oxalic acid, which can bind to calcium and form kidney stones in susceptible individuals. It's important to use rhubarb in moderation and to consult with a healthcare professional if you have any concerns or underlying health conditions.

Sarsaparilla:

Definition: Sarsaparilla refers to several species of plants belonging to the Smilax genus, including Smilax regelii and Smilax officinalis. It has been used historically in traditional medicine for its potential health benefits, particularly for its purported detoxifying and anti-inflammatory properties.

Ingredients: Sarsaparilla contains various bioactive compounds, including saponins (such as sarsaponin and smilagenin), flavonoids, phenolic acids, and sterols. These compounds are believed to contribute to the herb's medicinal properties, including its potential as a diuretic, blood purifier, and anti-inflammatory agent.

How to Prepare: Sarsaparilla root is typically prepared and consumed as an herbal tea, decoction, or tincture. To make tea, dried sarsaparilla root is steeped in hot water for several minutes before being strained and consumed. Decoctions involve boiling the root in water to extract its active compounds, while tinctures are prepared by steeping the root in alcohol or vinegar.

Dosage: The appropriate dosage of sarsaparilla can vary depending on factors such as age, health status, and the specific preparation being used. It's important to follow the recommended dosage on the product label or consult with a qualified herbalist or healthcare professional for personalized guidance.

How to Use: Sarsaparilla tea or tincture is typically taken orally. It's important to use sarsaparilla products as directed and to discontinue use if any adverse effects occur.

Side Effects: Sarsaparilla is generally considered safe for most people when used in moderate amounts. However, some individuals may experience allergic reactions or digestive upset. It may also interact with certain medications or have adverse effects in individuals with certain health conditions. It's important to use sarsaparilla under the guidance of a healthcare professional and to discontinue use if any adverse effects occur.

Wild Cherry Bark:

Definition: Wild cherry bark, scientifically known as Prunus serotina, is the bark obtained from the black cherry tree native to North America. It has been used traditionally in Native American and folk medicine for its potential health benefits, particularly for respiratory and digestive issues.

Ingredients: Wild cherry bark contains various bioactive compounds, including cyanogenic glycosides (such as prunasin and amygdalin), flavonoids, and phenolic acids. These compounds are believed to contribute to the herb's medicinal properties, including its potential as an expectorant, cough suppressant, and mild sedative.

How to Prepare: Wild cherry bark is typically prepared and consumed as an herbal tea, decoction, or syrup. To make tea, dried wild cherry bark is steeped in hot water for several minutes before being strained and consumed. Decoctions involve boiling the bark in water to extract its active compounds, while syrups are made by simmering the bark with sugar or honey to create a thick, sweet liquid.

Dosage: The appropriate dosage of wild cherry bark can vary depending on factors such as age, health status, and the specific preparation being used. It's important to follow the recommended dosage on the product label or consult with a qualified herbalist or healthcare professional for personalized guidance.

How to Use: Wild cherry bark tea, decoction, or syrup is typically taken orally. It's often consumed to soothe coughs, sore throats, and other respiratory symptoms. It's important to use wild cherry bark products as directed and to discontinue use if any adverse effects occur.

Side Effects: Wild cherry bark is generally considered safe for most people when used in moderate amounts. However, it contains cyanogenic glycosides, which can release cyanide in the body when metabolized. While the risk of cyanide poisoning from consuming wild cherry bark is low when used appropriately, excessive intake or prolonged use may lead to adverse effects. It's important to use wild cherry bark under the guidance of a healthcare professional and to discontinue use if any adverse effects occur.

Yellowdock:

Definition: Yellowdock, scientifically known as Rumex crispus, is a perennial flowering plant native to Europe and western Asia but is also found in North America. It has a long history of use in traditional medicine, particularly among Indigenous peoples, for its potential health benefits.

Ingredients: Yellowdock root contains various bioactive compounds, including anthraquinone glycosides (such as emodin and chrysophanol), tannins, and vitamins (including vitamin A and vitamin C). These compounds are believed to contribute to the herb's medicinal properties, including its potential as a laxative, blood cleanser, and liver tonic.

How to Prepare: Yellowdock root is typically prepared and consumed as an herbal tea, tincture, or capsule. To make tea, dried yellowdock root is steeped in hot water for several minutes before being strained and consumed. Tinctures are prepared by steeping the root in alcohol or vinegar to extract its active compounds.

Dosage: The appropriate dosage of yellowdock can vary depending on factors such as age, health status, and the specific preparation being used. It's important to follow the recommended dosage on the product label or consult with a qualified herbalist or healthcare professional for personalized guidance.

How to Use: Yellowdock tea, tincture, or capsules are typically taken orally. It's often consumed to support digestion, promote bowel regularity, and cleanse the blood. It's important to use yellowdock products as directed and to discontinue use if any adverse effects occur.

Side Effects: Yellowdock is generally considered safe for most people when used in moderate amounts. However, some individuals may experience mild side effects such as gastrointestinal upset or allergic reactions. It may also interact with certain medications or have adverse effects in individuals with certain health conditions. It's important to use yellowdock under the guidance of a healthcare professional and to discontinue use if any adverse effects occur.

Yellowdock Root:

Definition: Yellowdock root, scientifically known as Rumex crispus, is the root of a perennial flowering plant native to Europe and western Asia, also found in North America. It has a long history of use in traditional medicine, particularly among Indigenous peoples, for its potential health benefits.

Ingredients: Yellowdock root contains various bioactive compounds, including anthraquinone glycosides (such as emodin and chrysophanol), tannins, and vitamins (including vitamin A and vitamin C). These compounds are believed to contribute to the herb's medicinal properties, including its potential as a laxative, blood cleanser, and liver tonic.

How to Prepare: Yellowdock root is typically prepared and consumed as an herbal tea, tincture, or capsule. To make tea, dried yellowdock root is steeped in hot water for several minutes before being strained and consumed. Tinctures are prepared by steeping the root in alcohol or vinegar to extract its active compounds.

Dosage: The appropriate dosage of yellowdock root can vary depending on factors such as age, health status, and the specific preparation being used. It's important to follow the recommended dosage on the product label or consult with a qualified herbalist or healthcare professional for personalized guidance.

How to Use: Yellowdock root tea, tincture, or capsules are typically taken orally. It's often consumed to support digestion, promote bowel regularity, and cleanse the blood. It's important to use yellowdock root products as directed and to discontinue use if any adverse effects occur.

Side Effects: Yellowdock root is generally considered safe for most people when used in moderate amounts. However, some individuals may experience mild side effects such as gastrointestinal upset or allergic reactions. It may also interact with certain medications or have adverse effects in individuals with certain health conditions. It's important to use yellowdock root under the guidance of a healthcare professional and to discontinue use if any adverse effects occur.

Agrimony:

Definition: Agrimony, scientifically known as Agrimonia eupatoria, is a perennial herbaceous plant native to Europe, Asia, and North America. It has a long history of use in traditional medicine, particularly in European folk medicine, for its potential health benefits.

Ingredients: Agrimony contains various bioactive compounds, including tannins, flavonoids, phenolic acids, and volatile oils. These compounds are believed to contribute to the herb's medicinal properties, including its potential as an astringent, anti-inflammatory, and digestive aid.

How to Prepare: Agrimony is typically prepared and consumed as an herbal tea, tincture, or poultice. To make tea, dried agrimony leaves and flowers are steeped in hot water for several minutes before being strained and consumed. Tinctures are prepared by steeping the herb in alcohol or vinegar to extract its active compounds.

Dosage: The appropriate dosage of agrimony can vary depending on factors such as age, health status, and the specific preparation being used. It's important to follow the recommended dosage on the product label or consult with a qualified herbalist or healthcare professional for personalized guidance.

How to Use: Agrimony tea, tincture, or poultice is typically taken orally or applied topically. It's often consumed to soothe gastrointestinal issues, such as indigestion and diarrhea, or used externally to treat skin conditions.

Side Effects: Agrimony is generally considered safe for most people when used in moderate amounts. However, some individuals may experience allergic reactions or gastrointestinal upset. It may also interact with certain medications or have adverse effects in individuals with certain health conditions. It's important to use agrimony under the guidance of a healthcare professional and to discontinue use if any adverse effects occur.

Alfalfa:

Definition: Alfalfa, scientifically known as Medicago sativa, is a flowering plant in the pea family native to Asia but cultivated worldwide. It's primarily grown as fodder for livestock, but it has also been used in traditional medicine for its potential health benefits.

Ingredients: Alfalfa contains various bioactive compounds, including vitamins (such as vitamin A, vitamin C, and vitamin K), minerals (including calcium, magnesium, and potassium), amino acids, and phytoestrogens. These compounds are believed to contribute to the herb's medicinal properties, including its potential as a nutritive tonic, diuretic, and hormone balancer.

How to Prepare: Alfalfa is typically consumed as sprouts, herbal tea, or in supplement form (such as capsules or tablets). To make tea, dried alfalfa leaves are steeped in hot water for several minutes before being strained and consumed.

Dosage: The appropriate dosage of alfalfa can vary depending on factors such as age, health status, and the specific preparation being used. It's important to follow the recommended dosage on the product label or consult with a qualified herbalist or healthcare professional for personalized guidance.

How to Use: Alfalfa sprouts, tea, or supplements are typically taken orally. It's often consumed as a dietary supplement to support overall health and well-being, as well as to promote kidney health and hormone balance.

Side Effects: Alfalfa is generally considered safe for most people when consumed in moderate amounts. However, some individuals may experience allergic reactions or digestive upset. It may also interact with certain medications or have adverse effects in individuals with certain health conditions, such as autoimmune diseases or hormone-sensitive conditions. Pregnant or breastfeeding individuals should consult with a healthcare professional before using alfalfa supplements. It's important to use alfalfa under the guidance of a healthcare professional and to discontinue use if any adverse effects occur.

Ashwagandha:

Definition: Ashwagandha, scientifically known as Withaniasomnifera, is a small shrub native to India, the Middle East, and parts of Africa. It has a long history of use in Ayurvedic medicine for its potential health benefits, particularly for its adaptogenic properties.

Ingredients: Ashwagandha root contains various bioactive compounds, including alkaloids (such as withanolides), steroidal lactones, and flavonoids. These compounds are believed to contribute to the herb's medicinal properties, including its potential as an adaptogen, anti-inflammatory, and immune-modulating agent.

How to Prepare: Ashwagandha is typically consumed as a powdered root, herbal tea, tincture, or in supplement form (such as capsules or tablets). To make tea, dried ashwagandha root is steeped in hot water for several minutes before being strained and consumed.

Dosage: The appropriate dosage of ashwagandha can vary depending on factors such as age, health status, and the specific preparation being used. It's important to follow the recommended dosage on the product label or consult with a qualified herbalist or healthcare professional for personalized guidance.

How to Use: Ashwagandha powder, tea, tincture, or supplements are typically taken orally. It's often consumed to support stress management, promote relaxation, and boost overall vitality and well-being.

Side Effects: Ashwagandha is generally considered safe for most people when used in moderate amounts. However, some individuals may experience mild side effects such as gastrointestinal upset or drowsiness. It may also interact with certain medications or have adverse effects in individuals with certain health conditions, such as autoimmune diseases or thyroid disorders. Pregnant or breastfeeding individuals should consult with a healthcare professional before using ashwagandha supplements. It's important to use ashwagandha under the guidance of a healthcare professional and to discontinue use if any adverse effects occur.

Black Cohosh:

Definition: Black cohosh, scientifically known as Actaea racemosa (formerly Cimicifuga racemosa), is a perennial herb native to North America. It has a long history of use in traditional Native American medicine and later in folk medicine for its potential health benefits, particularly for women's health.

Ingredients: Black cohosh root contains various bioactive compounds, including triterpene glycosides (such as actein and cimicifugoside), phenolic acids, and flavonoids. These compounds are believed to contribute to the herb's medicinal properties, including its potential as a hormone-balancing agent and its ability to relieve menopausal symptoms.

How to Prepare: Black cohosh is typically consumed as a powdered root, herbal tea, tincture, or in supplement form (such as capsules or tablets). To make tea, dried black cohosh root is steeped in hot water for several minutes before being strained and consumed.

Dosage: The appropriate dosage of black cohosh can vary depending on factors such as age, health status, and the specific preparation being used. It's important to follow the recommended dosage on the product label or consult with a qualified herbalist or healthcare professional for personalized guidance.

How to Use: Black cohosh powder, tea, tincture, or supplements are typically taken orally. It's often used by women to support hormonal balance, relieve menopausal symptoms such as hot flashes and night sweats, and promote overall well-being.

Side Effects: Black cohosh is generally considered safe for most people when used in moderate amounts. However, some individuals may experience mild side effects such as gastrointestinal upset or allergic reactions. It may also interact with certain medications or have adverse effects in individuals with certain health conditions, such as liver disease or hormone-sensitive conditions. Pregnant or breastfeeding individuals should consult with a healthcare professional before using black cohosh supplements. It's important to use black cohosh under the guidance of a healthcare professional and to discontinue use if any adverse effects occur.

Tila:

Definition: Tila, also known as linden flower or lime blossom, refers to the flowers of the Tilia genus, primarily Tilia europaea and Tilia cordata. These trees are native to Europe, but they are also cultivated in other regions for their fragrant and medicinal flowers.

Ingredients: Tila flowers contain various bioactive compounds, including flavonoids, phenolic acids, and volatile oils. These compounds are believed to contribute to the herb's medicinal properties, including its potential as a mild sedative, anxiolytic, and anti-inflammatory agent.

How to Prepare: Tila flowers are typically prepared and consumed as an herbal tea or infusion. To make tea, dried tila flowers are steeped in hot water for several minutes before being strained and consumed.

Dosage: The appropriate dosage of tila can vary depending on factors such as age, health status, and the specific preparation being used. It's important to follow the recommended dosage on the product label or consult with a qualified herbalist or healthcare professional for personalized guidance.

How to Use: Tila tea is typically taken orally. It's often consumed in the evening as a calming bedtime beverage or during times of stress or anxiety. It's important to use tila products as directed and to discontinue use if any adverse effects occur.

Side Effects: Tila is generally considered safe for most people when used in moderate amounts. However, some individuals may experience allergic reactions or digestive upset. It may also interact with certain medications or have adverse effects in individuals with certain health conditions. It's important to use tila under the guidance of a healthcare professional and to discontinue use if any adverse effects occur.

Valerian:

Definition: Valerian, scientifically known as Valeriana officinalis, is a perennial flowering plant native to Europe and Asia. It has been used for centuries in traditional medicine for its potential calming and sedative effects.

Ingredients: Valerian root contains several bioactive compounds, including valerenic acid, valepotriates, and volatile oils. These compounds are believed to contribute to the herb's medicinal properties, including its potential as a sedative, anxiolytic, and sleep aid.

How to Prepare: Valerian root is typically prepared and consumed as an herbal tea, tincture, or capsule. To make tea, dried valerian root is steeped in hot water for several minutes before being strained and consumed. Tinctures are prepared by steeping the root in alcohol or vinegar to extract its active compounds.

Dosage: The appropriate dosage of valerian can vary depending on factors such as age, health status, and the specific preparation being used. It's important to follow the recommended dosage on the product label or consult with a qualified herbalist or healthcare professional for personalized guidance.

How to Use: Valerian tea, tincture, or capsules are typically taken orally. It's often consumed in the evening as a sleep aid or during times of stress or anxiety. It's important to use valerian products as directed and to discontinue use if any adverse effects occur.

Side Effects: Valerian is generally considered safe for most people when used in moderate amounts. However, some individuals may experience mild side effects such as drowsiness, headache, or gastrointestinal upset. It may also interact with certain medications or have adverse effects in individuals with certain health conditions. It's important to use valerian under the guidance of a healthcare professional and to discontinue use if any adverse effects occur.

Guaco:

Definition: Guaco, also known as Mikania cordata or Mikania glomerata, is a medicinal plant native to Central and South America. It has a long history of use in traditional medicine for its potential therapeutic properties.

Ingredients: Guaco contains several bioactive compounds, including coumarins, flavonoids, tannins, and saponins. These compounds are believed to contribute to the herb's medicinal properties, including its potential as an expectorant, anti-inflammatory, and antispasmodic agent.

How to Prepare: Guaco is typically prepared and consumed as an herbal tea or infusion. To make tea, dried guaco leaves are steeped in hot water for several minutes before being strained and consumed.

Dosage: The appropriate dosage of guaco can vary depending on factors such as age, health status, and the specific preparation being used. It's important to follow the recommended dosage on the product label or consult with a qualified herbalist or healthcare professional for personalized guidance.

How to Use: Guaco tea is typically taken orally. It can be consumed on its own or mixed with honey or other herbal teas for added flavor.

Side Effects: Guaco is generally considered safe for most people when used in moderate amounts. However, some individuals may experience allergic reactions or digestive upset. It may also interact with certain medications or have adverse effects in individuals with certain health conditions. It's important to use guaco under the guidance of a healthcare professional and to discontinue use if any adverse effects occur.

THE END